C000088531

Healing
Back Pain

with Osteopathic Tension Releasing Exercises

About the book

A functioning self-healing and immune system can solve virtually any health problem. Therefore osteopathy focuses on activating these oftentimes impaired self-healing powers and thereby achieve a completely natural healing. The cause of impaired self-healing powers is a problem with the nourishing and cleansing of the cells, the muscles, the bones or any other structure. The osteopath achieves this by means of his knowledge of human anatomy and physiology and with finesse of his palpation. The osteopathic techniques are however also wonderfully suited for self-treatment. This is where personal body-awareness comes into play.

In this book, Thomas Seebeck conveys the principles of osteopathic treatment, and a variety of exercises for healing back pain at all areas of the spine. The exercises are illustrated in a detailed and practical manner.

This book is a subset of the book "Osteopathic Self-Treatment" written by the same author.

About the author

Thomas Seebeck, born 1971, has been a physiotherapist since 1995 and has been running his own clinic in Dinklage (Germany) since 2002. In 2006 he received the Diploma in Osteopathic Therapy from the German Society of Osteopathic Medicine (DGOM), for which he has also been a teacher since 2008. He is the chairman of the German Association for Osteopathic Therapy (DAGOT) and academician of the DGOM.

He dedicates his free time to music, amongst other things, classic Chinese medicine, and QiGong and loves windsurfing. He runs mindfulness courses together with his brother, Andreas.

Thomas Seebeck

Healing
Back Pain

with Osteopathic
Tension Releasing
Exercises

LOTUS PRESS

Important advice: the methods and suggestions in this book represent the author's opinion and experience. They were compiled according to the best of his knowledge and were tested as carefully as possible. They are not, however, a substitute for competent medical advice. The reader is personally responsible for his actions. Neither the author, nor the publishing company can be held accountable for any negative side effects or damages resulting from following the practical suggestions provided in this book.

Thomas Seebeck
Healing Back Pain with Osteopathic Tension Releasing Exercises

Copyright by Lotus-Press, 2015
Layout: Andreas Seebeck
Additional images used under license from Shutterstock.com

All rights, particularly the right of reproduction of any kind, including via electronic media, and the translation into other languages, are reserved. No reproduction, not even partial reproduction, is permitted without the publisher's consent.

All rights reserved.

www.lotus-press.com

ISBN 978-3-945430-28-6

For Kerstin

Contents

Appraisal for osteopathic self-treatment exercises

It is empowering to have a set of exercises at hand to take care of your body.

Light Within Enterprises

I have used many of the exercises for the head and neck to help with the management of a chronic neurologic disorder. I have noticed that the frequency of symptoms has decreased and discussed this also with my neurologist. He is happy with the results also and has suggested I continue using the exercises[].

Rachael Monaco

... try each exercise. I already feel better!!

Alicia McIntyre

I recommend this to anyone because it helped me control my headaches I usually have.

Tiffany G.

We as a family have tried a few of these and I will tell you they truly work. Thank you so much for sharing the knowledge.

Jennifer

I have asked a few questions pertaining to organic action and life, because Nature is a school of question and answers, which seems to be the only school in which man learns anything.

A.T. Still

Introduction

Sit in an upright and relaxed position on a chair or stool. Take a moment and feel the air flowing through your nostrils.

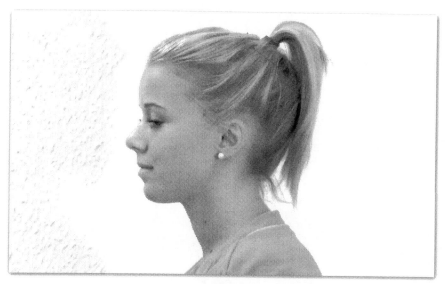

The three components of the exercises: breathing, movement and awareness.

Discern carefully: does more air flow through the right or left nostril or is the difference unnoticeable? Can you feel that the air you breathe out is warmer than the air you breathe in?

Now guide your awareness to your torso and spine. Can you sense that your breathing is connected with a small movement of your torso and spine? When you breathe in, your spine extends a little, and when you breathe out it retracts a little. If you can sense this, then you are ready for your self-treatment, because for this you will not require much more than a sense of breathing and movement.

Your first osteopathic self-treatment

In the introduction I asked you to feel the connection between breathing in and the slight extension of the spine, and breathing out and the slight bending of the spine. Now please try to find out which direction of movement is more comfortable for you. If you cannot be sure with very small movements, simply make the movements larger. Please remember though, that you are trying to find the maximum relaxation. If you move too far into the more comfortable position, the tension increases again.

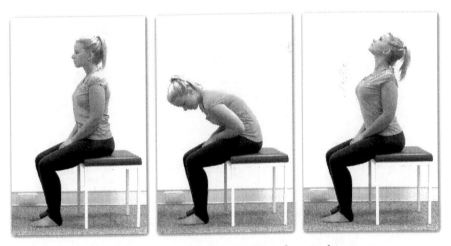

Testing: neutral, bending and stretching

Test

Bend forward only as far as it is comfortable. Be mindful of the feeling when returning to the neutral position. If it is uncomfortable, you have moved too far!

When stretching you will obviously reach your movement barrier much sooner. However if you move carefully and mindfully, this could be your more comfortable direction of movement.

Once you have found out which one of the two directions is more comfortable for you, combine this movement with breathing. There are two options.

If **stretching** is the more comfortable movement for you, then breathe in while moving into the comfortable position, and breathe out while returning to the neutral position.

Now switch the breathing around: breathe out as you stretch and breathe in while returning to the neutral position. Which combination feels better? If you cannot feel a difference, pick an exercise randomly.

If your more comfortable movement is **bending forward**, then breathe in while bending forward and breathe out while returning upwards. Then the other way around: breathe out while bending forward and breathe in while returning to the neutral position. Which combination feels better?

Exercise

Repeat your "comfortable combination" of breathing and movement for several breaths. It is reasonable to take a little break after breathing in and then out, i.e. to stop breathing and movement at the same time. The length of these breaks depends on what you feel is comfortable. After a while you will better be able to feel the impulse to continue breathing.

End the exercise after a maximum time of two minutes. Take a short break, in which you perhaps might briefly move your shoulders or shake yourself out a little.

Retest

First test the direction of movement that you exercised. Never mind the breathing now. This movement should at least not feel worse. Now test the other direction. Can you feel a change? Normally, this movement should now feel better than it did in the initial test. If this is the case, congratulations! You have just successfully completed your first osteopathic self-treatment.

If there is no improvement or you could not feel a difference in the movements in the beginning, you probably require a different direction of exercise. The principle of the exercise, however, remains the same.

Basically, if you can feel a difference, exercise the better option. That might seem strange at first, but once you have understood it and successfully put it into practice, it becomes really easy. Sooner or later you will find an exercise after which your discomforts will suddenly disappear. From that moment on, these exercises can become highly addictive, partly because you will suddenly have the feeling that you have recovered part of the responsibility for your own health and that you can do something straight away when you feel an ache or pain.

Crucial to success is that you perform the exercises mindfully, i.e. that you put your mind and heart into the exercises. In the beginning, the movements' amplitude should be large, so that energetic and structural blockades can be dissolved, muscle tensions can be relaxed and the strain hardening and immobilization of the smaller and larger vertebral joints can be mobilized. The movements of the spinal column and its smaller and larger joints have a traction-compression effect on the intervertebral discs. This traction-compression effect has a positive effect on the cartilage discs' elasticity, which can soak up with fluid again due to the movement's stimulus. Their elasticity allows them to better fulfill their buffering function.

Your movements should be

- steady, not abrupt

- round, not angular
- soft, not stiff
- slow, not hectic
- gentle, not forced.

The three planes of movement

The testing of movements is always performed on the basis of the three base planes of space, i.e. the body. The "yes plane" (sagittal plane) depicts bending and stretching movements, like e.g. nodding your head. The "no plane" (horizontal plane) depicts horizontal turning movements as e.g. performed when shaking your head. The "maybe plane" (frontal plane) depicts sideway movements, like e.g. the leaning of your head to the left and right.

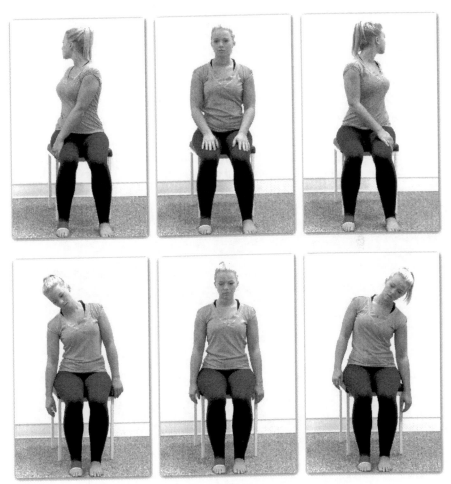

The "no plane" and the "maybe plane"

Overview of the exercise sequence

Test

Testing the movement: which is the more comfortable direction?
Testing the breathing: how does the breathing best match the more comfortable direction of movement? Does it feel more comfortable when

- you move in the better direction while breathing in and return to the middle while breathing out? Or
- when you move in the better direction while breathing out and return while breathing in?

Exercise

Repeat the "comfortable combination" of breathing and movement for several breaths or minutes. After breathing in and out, stop breathing and movement at the same time.

Retest

Retest the movement first to the better, and then to the worse side. Be aware of the difference to the initial test.

Part 1: Osteopathic Principles

Unlike you would think

When I was 17 years old I attended "Tae-Kwon-Do" martial arts classes twice a week. The training was tough and pushed me to my breaking point. And yet I never had sore muscles, except on two occasions. Due to other commitments I had to leave training early and the next day my calve muscles ached. The part of training I had missed out on, was the short meditation, sitting seiza style. In this position a large part of the calve- muscles are in maximum approximation and relaxation.

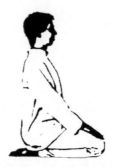

Sitting seiza-style

I did not realize at that point, that this was my first osteopathic self-treatment according to the principle of the "indirect technique", but I never forgot it.

Key principles of osteopathy

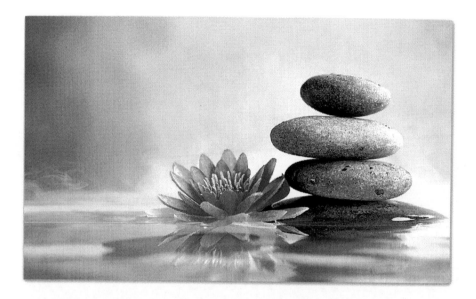

A functioning self-healing and immune system can solve virtually any health problem. Therefore osteopathy focuses on activating these oftentimes impaired self-healing powers and thereby achieve a completely natural healing.

Direct and indirect technique

In osteopathy we generally deal with two opposing directions. If we move towards a barrier, we call it the "direct technique" (directly towards the barrier). Imagine working as a waiter and carrying a dinner tray with heavy plates and glasses all day long. If you are not used to this strain, by the evening you are not able to stretch your arm properly and you feel as if your elbow were out of joint. However, if you anyway try to stretch your arm, you are working towards the barrier, i.e. with the direct technique. If you move your arm away from this barrier by bending it, so that it can relax optimally, you are applying the indirect technique. Yoga's stretching exercises correspond, from an osteopathic viewpoint, to the direct technique, whereby Yoga obviously is more than simply a stretching exercise program. Just as with all movement meditations (Qigong, Taijiquan, etc.), inner guidance of movement plays a large role with yoga and osteopathy.

The indirect technique is particularly employed in osteopathy in the case of heavy pain and large problems, because in this relieving position/direction the nourishment of the affected tissue is improved. Imagine trying to water a dry bed with a bent water hose. Moving into the position of maximum relaxation is like straightening out the bend in the hose, so that the exchange of substances can continue unhindered. In self-treatment this movement/position is mostly the more comfortable one, the "comfortable direction". To find out which one it is, you have to test both directions.

Key principles of osteopathy

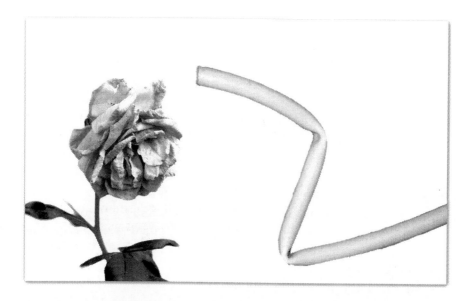

The cause of impaired self-healing powers is a problem with the nourishing and cleansing of the cells, the muscles, the bones or any other structure.

Direct and indirect technique in nature

"We believe the reason of this great absence of disease among animals and fowls of all kinds was a strict adherence to the laws under which they were placed by Nature. When they were tired the would rest, when hungry they would eat, and lived in strict obedience to all the indications of their wants. We believe man is not an exception to this rule."

A.T. Still

We can find many examples of the "indirect technique" in nature. A dog will always keep his damaged paw in a position of maximum relaxation and will lie down in a corner so that it can heal ("indirect technique"). Every now and again he will try to walk normally ("direct technique"). Once this is possible, he resumes normal walking. This is our inborn, human behavior. For example, when our stomach hurts, we bend over double, in order to allow the stomach muscles and the underlying tissue to relax optimally.

However with chronic or minor discomforts, we often suppress this natural behavior and even try to cause more tension, possibly even forcibly, along the lines of "there has to be a way!". Afterwards we wonder why our discomfort has intensified. I like to compare this behavior with a jammed door lock. Trying to open it by force will simply cause it to jam even more. However, if you gently push the lock ("indirect technique), it opens easily.

23

Key principles of osteopathy

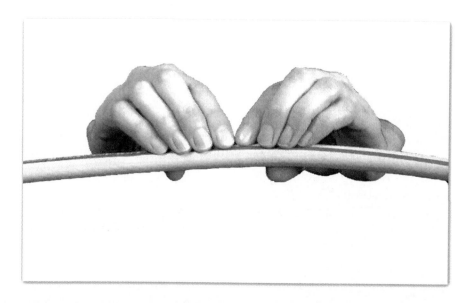

The osteopath avails himself of his profound knowledge of human anatomy and physiology, as well as finesse of his palpation to detect and do away with these problems related to nourishment and cleansing. In the case of self-treatment, your own body awareness is more than enough.

Osteopathy – supporting nature's healing powers

Andrew Taylor Still, MD, DO (1828 – 1917) was the founder of osteopathy and osteopathic medicine. He was also a physician and sur-
geon, author, inventor and the founder of the American School of Osteopathy (now A.T. Still University), the world's first osteopathic
medical school, in Kirksville, Missouri. Dr. Still kept emphasizing,
that it was the osteopath's job to find health, not illness. After all,
anyone could find illness. The stance, the principle fundamental to
osteopathy, is that we should focus on the aspect of "nature's healing
powers". Instead of fighting illness (as a principle), we try to put the
body in a position that enables healing. Try to integrate the following
aspect into your thinking: when you feel ill, you already bear the seed
of recovery inside yourself. This seed can grow faster, if you concentrate on your well-being instead of on fighting an illness.

"Activating Forces"

The conscious use of breathing is a so-called "activating force", os-
teopathically seen, i.e. an activating power. Activating forces make
an exercise more effective, or really effective in the first place. Other
activating forces are

- Emotions. You can put yourself in a certain emotional condi-
tion while performing the exercise. For example, how about
closing your eyes and imagining yourself on a warm beach in
the South Pacific, on a six-week holiday?

- Oscillations (vibrations). Shaking ("tou") has been known in
all Qigong traditions for thousands of years. It should be used,
preferably, in the breathing pauses. If you have detected on
the "yes plane" that bowing your head is more comfortable
than stretching it, lightly and effortlessly shake your head in
the holding position.

- Stacking. All three planes of movement are adjusted one after the other, so that the maximum comfort is reached. They are "stacked". You can, e.g. test whether it is easier to turn your head to the left or to the right ("no plane"), then in the comfortable position you add a small movement from the "yes plane", and finally a minimal movement from the "maybe plane". From plane to plane the movements become ever smaller, because the maneuvering room decreases.

- Own muscle strength. With some exercises you work with your own muscle strength (e.g. the exercise "pelvic area" – hip joint/pubic bone/adductors).

If you are not yet satisfied with the outcome of the exercises, simply try to employ further activating forces when performing the exercises.

Strain-Counterstrain (SCS)

The American physician and osteopath Dr. Jones developed the strain-counterstrain technique in the 1960s for the purpose of treating pain. It is based on the principle of wrapping tissue, i.e. the body around the painful point, as one for example does when bending over double in the case of stomach pain. The technique was slightly adapted, so that it can be used in self-treatment.

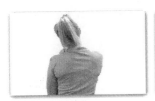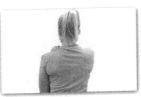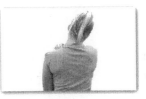

Pressure-sensitive pain points can be treated excellently with the strain-counterstrain technique

Test

If you have a point on your body that is painful under pressure, this technique is extremely useful. These are mostly found in the neck muscles. Use your right-hand fingers to find such a point on the left side of your neck.

Did you find such a pain point? Touch it so you feel a slight (!) pain in order to perform the movement tests.

Test the cervical spine on the "maybe plane". The pain probably will reduce when you tilt your head to the affected side. Leave your head like that and adjust it on the "yes-" and "no level" so that the pain possibly even disappears.

Exercise

Breathe in and out several times, consciously aware of that point, while maintaining it pain free. According to Dr Jones, it completely suffices to hold the pain point for one and a half to two minutes. Discontinue the exercise if it causes discomfort. Afterwards return to the starting position.

Retest

Take a short break, maybe shaking out your shoulders, and then retest the painful point. The pain should have reduced significantly (at least by 70%).

The "onion of discomfort"

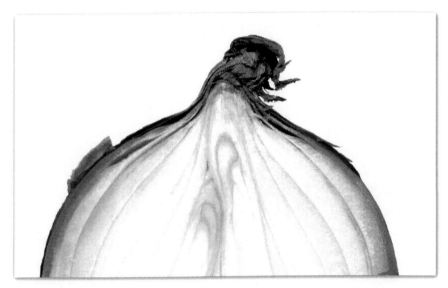

Sometimes osteopathic self-treatment is like peeling an onion

Many patients wonder why, after an osteopathic treatment of e.g. the knee, the pain in their neck is reduced. This happens all the time in osteopathy. The osteopath knows that "pain is a great liar" and therefore searches for the actual cause of discomfort.

Example: A person is in an accident and his left knee is injured. After a while this leads to often unnoticed changes in his gait. The body is constantly seeking balance (compensation). Due to its capability of compensation, e.g. through the pelvis muscles, no discomfort is felt and therefore no physician is consulted. At some point another injury is sustained, maybe on the shoulder or head. Once again the body tried to balance the tensions. If the two compensations oppose each other, this causes discomfort in the neck, where two teams are playing "tug of war". The osteopath can find the trouble-causing knee or shoulder. But based on the principle of the "onion of discomfort", the patient can find the hidden cause of discomfort. In this example that means that although the neck is in pain and can therefore be called the area of the "tug of war", it is not the cause of discomfort. After a successful self-treatment of this area, the knee or shoulder will emerge as the cause of discomfort. After further self-treatment of that problem area, the discomforts should disappear permanently.

This is why osteopathy often speaks of "linkage syndrome". All the body's structures, down to the individual cell, are interlinked. We are not cars or machines made up of assembled spare parts. So it should not surprise you if discomforts wander through your body. This is often simply due to the linkage patterns of your body. If you are aware of your body and exercise it mindfully, you will soon feel that not just one particular discomfort disappears, but rather, that your movements become lighter and freer because your body's tensile stress is better distributed.

Be open to any changes that can result from the exercises, but do not expect miracles. Some discomforts disappear immediately. But you might feel a pain in another spot or you might remember something suppressed or forgotten. Clearly perceive it and decide whether it might belong to the discomfort, which lead you to perform the exercise. Your body can give you more clues to lead you to a healthier, happier life than you might think. You just need to learn to listen.

We tend to avoid taking a closer look at problems because they scare us. Fear means stress, and stress blocks the part of the vegetative nervous system responsible for healing (parasympathetic nervous system). The exercises will help you to regain your trust in nature's healing power (A.T. Still) because you no longer will be at the mercy of your discomforts. The more discomforts your have, the easier it will be for you to find the corresponding exercise, because your body gives you clear signals that something is not right.

Part 2: Exercises from top to bottom

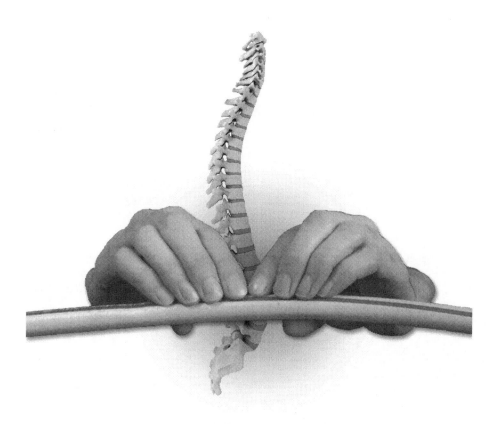

"The body of man [is] God's drug-store and [has] in it all liquids, drugs, lubricating oils, opiates, acids, and anti-acids, and every sort of drug that the wisdom of God thought necessary for human happiness and health."

A.T. Still

Dr. Still warned of a recipe-like, i.e. technical approach to osteopathy. You may adapt each exercise to your feeling. Only maintain the basic structure of "test, exercise, retest".

Note: The illustrated exercises are the result of more than 20 years of collaboration with my patients. I was constantly searching with them for the fitting exercise and each one had to be individually adapted because no two people are the same. So I cannot promise you that "your" exercise is among these. But once you have understood the principle, you will easily find your own self-treatment options. Be playful and curious. The exercises should always be interesting and pleasant, never boring, uncomfortable or exhausting. I promise you, if you perform the exercises with awareness, you will always perceive changes.

In the words of A.T. Still,

"Now make yourself a child of inquiry and a student of Nature."

Cervical spine

The tissue at the area of the cervical spine is considered a crucial point that benefits from strengthening, both in Eastern and Western medicine. It needs to be kept relaxed and properly aligned as the first step to proper posture. Within the bony casing located directly at the juncture of the skull and the first spinal vertebra lies the terminal nerve bundle of the spinal cord as it leads into the base of the brain. Tightness or obstruction will restrict the blood flow and nerve impulses to and from the brain. Misalignment at the very top vertebra can result in overcompensation in the position of the jaw, the muscles of the face, and along the length of the spine, which leads to poor posture, pain, and fatigue. In time, more serious conditions such as bone spurs, disk problems, and compromised immune function can develop if not addressed.

A properly aligned spine results in a healthy nervous system, which in turn elevates all other functions of the body. A healthy neck is very important for total well-being. Use the following exercises to keep it open and aligned in order for the nerve impulses to properly flow to and from the brain. Bodily functions, such as breathing and blood pressure, are controlled from the brain stem. Any degeneration here will negatively affect the body over time. A stiff neck will lead to all sorts of pain in the body and head. A loose, flexible neck will improve your overall health.

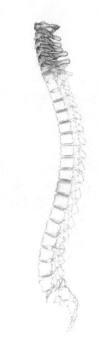

The cervical spine

Discomforts at the back of your head (upper cervical spine)

Discomforts at the back of your head often are related to dysfunctions of the upper cervical spine. So you will find the corresponding exercises in the chapter "cervical spine". The following exercise, loosely based on an exercise by Dr. Robert Fulford, can be performed sitting, standing or lying on your back.

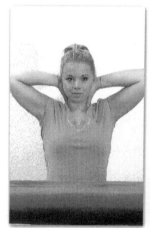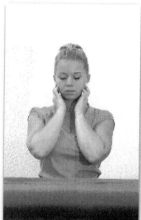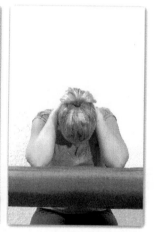

From left to right: exercise without support, feeling out the mastoid process, exercise with support

Test

Interlace your fingers and place your head in your hands so that the thenars (balls of your thumbs) touch the mastoid processes (the humps you can feel behind your ear) of the temporal bones. Gently pull the tissue of this area upwards with your thenars whilst you lower your head. Then do it the opposite way around. Lift your head and pull the tissue around the mastoid processes down. Once you have detected the more comfortable direction, combine it with breathing. Is the movement better performed while breathing in or out?

Exercise

Perform the combination of breathing and movement for one to two minutes. Be gentle and very careful. The most common mistake with this exercise is pushing or pulling too hard.

Retest

Retest both directions of movement and be aware of any changes.

Cervical spine

The main exercise in cases of discomforts in the cervical spine area is performed on the "yes-", "no-" and "maybe plane".

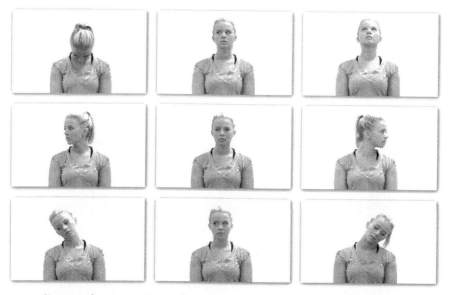

Cervical spine, "yes plane", "no plane", "maybe plane"

Test

Test which one of the following six directions of movement you perceive as most comfortable:

- Bending your head forward/stretching it back ("yes plane")
- Turning your head to the right/to the left ("no plane")
- Tilting your head towards the right shoulder/towards the left shoulder ("maybe plane")

Which of the six directions feels most comfortable? Combine it with breathing. Is the movement performed better while breathing in or out?

Exercise

Perform the most comfortable combination of breathing and movement for one to two minutes.

Retest

Retest all six directions and be aware of any changes.

For the upper cervical spine, especially in the area of the head joints, it is very useful if the movements are only minimal, as if giving a secret sign. Sometimes even just moving the eyes is sufficient.

Discomforts in the neck radiating into the head (cervical spine)

The cervical spine is an area of pain that often stems from a completely different area. It is most important for our body to keep its eye level perfectly balanced. So if a maladjustment in the pelvic area causes the eye level to be off-balance, the cervical spine automatically compensates, which can cause discomforts. If problems keep on arising in the cervical spine area and the exercises do not provide lasting relief, note in which other body areas you sense discomfort (onion of discomfort). Applying osteopathic self-treatment to the corresponding area should reduce the discomforts in the cervical spine area as well.

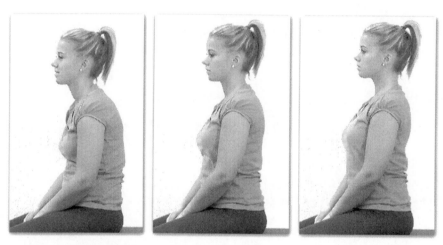

The balloon/lead-weight exercise requires some imagination

Test

Sit upright and relaxed on a chair or a stool. Make sure you have a straight posture. You might have to lift the tip of your sternum by one or two centimeters, in order to better balance your head on your cervical spine (as one would a ball on a vertical rod). Imagine your head to be light, wanting to float upwards, like a helium-filled balloon.

Now imagine your head to be as heavy as lead and your cervical spine sinking under that weight.

Test both directions without prejudice. Sometimes the "lead-head" is more comfortable, even though the "light head" sounds better.

Once you have determined the more comfortable direction, combine it with breathing. Is it better combined with breathing in or breathing out?

Exercise

Perform the combination of breathing and movement for one to two minutes.

Retest

Retest both directions of movement and be aware of any changes.

Thoracic spine

By twisting and bending the spine, you are squeezing out the damp-ness that accumulates in the body like wringing the water out of a wet towel. You are creating this nourishing and dispersing movement on all the points along the spine. The benefit of this exercises is all in the right movement. It is not important how far you can stretch, but rather how smoothly you can move.

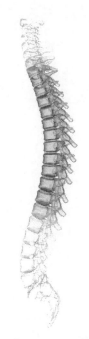

The thoracic spine

The area of the thoracic spine/chest/ribs – sitting down

Begin with the easiest exercises.

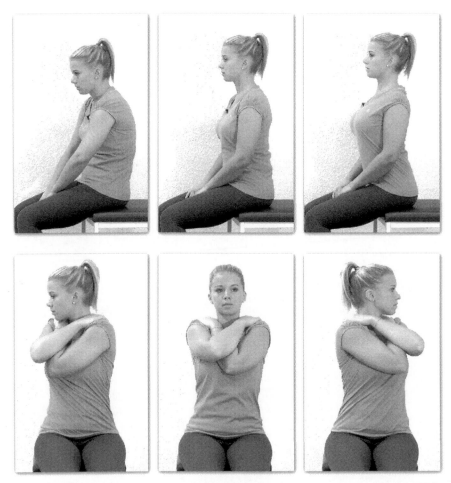

Testing the spine: above "yes plane", below "no plane"

Test

Test which one of the following six directions of movement is the most comfortable to you:

- Bending your thoracic spine forwards/ stretching it backwards ("yes plane")
- Turning the thoracic spine to the right/to the left ("no plane")
- Tilting the thoracic spine to the right/to the left ("maybe plane")

Which of the six directions is the most comfortable to you? Combine it with breathing. Is it easier to perform the movement while breathing in or out?

Exercise

Perform this combination for one to two minutes.

Retest

Retest all six directions of movement and be aware of any changes.

The area of the thoracic spine/chest/ribs – standing

The following option, performed while standing, is particularly effective. Keep your feet apart at shoulder width, your knees slightly bent. Lay your hands on the opposite shoulder and bend over slightly, so that you can feel a comfortable pull.

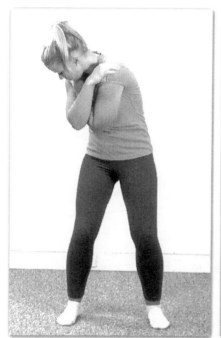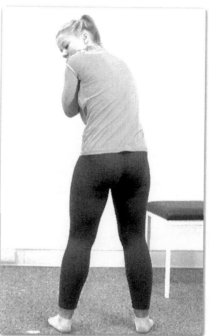

The "no plane" in a standing position

Test

Turn your torso left/right.

Have you determined the more comfortable direction? Then you just have to find out what breathing matches it best.

Exercise

Perform the combination of breathing and movement for two to three minutes.

Retest

Retest both movements and be aware of any changes.

The counterstrain exercise for the chest area

This exercise is useful e.g. for pain in the area of the thoracic spine, the ribs and the sternum. But it can also be helpful for discomforts caused by inner organs, e.g. acid reflux.

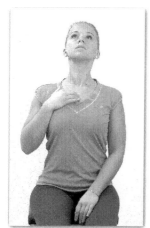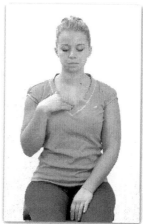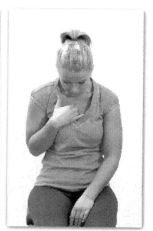

With the strain-counterstrain technique, be mindful of changes of the pain point while testing the planes

Test

Locate the pain point in the area of the sternum and the rib edges. Then test the effect of moving the spine on all three planes, one after the other. Begin by testing the bending and stretching of the upper body ("yes plane"). More often the bending leads to pain reduction. Remain in the most comfortable position. From there test on the "no plane", i.e. turn your upper body left and right and once again remain in the most comfortable position. Finally add tilting your body ("maybe plane"). The movements' amplitude keeps getting smaller with this exercise. Once you found the optimal position, the pain of the pain point should be reduced to 20% or less. The positioning of your body works best if you imagine you are wrapping yourself around the pain point.

Exercise

While maintaining the most pain free position, and holding the point with your finger, breathe in and out relaxed. Make sure that your finger pressure is gentle and not causing any pain. It might be useful to increase and decrease the pressure either while breathing in or out – try it and follow your feeling. Perform the exercise for at least two minutes. In this time you can fine-tune your position.

Retest

Slowly return to the initial position and retest the pain point. The pain should be reduced by at least 70%. Ideally you should not be able to trigger it at that point.

Lumbar spine

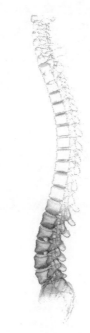

The lumbar spine

Exercise with stronger back pain

If the pain is stronger, it is recommended to perform the exercise in a position that is as pain-free as possible. For the sternum and the lumbar spine this is often the all-fours position. You can test all three planes from this position and perform the corresponding exercise.

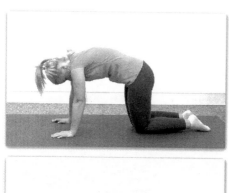

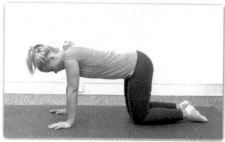

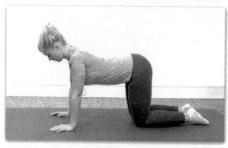

When nothing else works: the all-fours position, here the test in the "yes plane"

Test

- Bend/stretch the thoracic spine ("yes plane")
- Turn the thoracic spine to the right/to the left ("no plane")
- Tilt the thoracic spine to the right/left side ("maybe plane")

Which of the six directions feels most comfortable? Combine it with breathing. Is the movement better performed while breathing in or out?

If the movements on the "no-" and "maybe plane" are too complicated for you, simply exercise on the "yes plane".

Exercise

Perform the combination of breathing and movement for two to three minutes.

Retest

Retest the movements on the exercise plane and be aware of any changes.

Discomforts of the lumbar spine

Discomforts of the lumbar spine can often be very persistent and tend to become chronic. When asking patients how long they have suffered of these discomforts, they often answer "forever". One reason for this, that is oftentimes overlooked, is that they are not dealing with a case of limited mobility, but rather of excess mobility or instability.

The following exercises are for limited mobility.

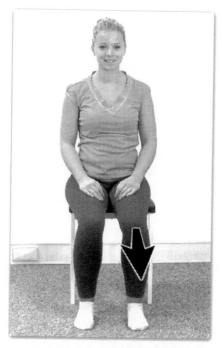

"No plane": if you push one knee forward, the pelvis turns in the corresponding direction

Test

Sit in an upright and relaxed position on a chair or a stool. Now push your right knee one to three centimeters forward, so that your pelvis begins to turn ("no plane"). Return to the original position and test the same movement with your left knee. Have you detected the more comfortable direction of movement? Now all you have to do, is find out which breathing phase best matches the movement.

Exercise

Perform the combination of breathing and movement for approximately two minutes.

Retest

Retest both movements and be aware of any changes.

While performing the exercise in the "yes plane", i.e. when bending and stretching the lumbar spine, it is helpful to imagine your pelvis being a bowl full of water. Move your pelvis as if you were carefully pouring water to the front and to the back. When tilting to the side, press one of the ischial tuberosities into the seat and imagine, viewed from the front, your lumbar spine forming a "C".

Exercises for the whole spine

How do the exercises work?

In everyday life the spinal column is mostly exposed to smaller and larger strains. Most people have fixed sections, often including several vertebrae, which cause discomforts. The related muscles are tense and often form myogelosis (hardening of the muscles). The spinal column's movements have a mobilizing effect on all the structures related to the spinal column. Vertebrae and costovertebral joints with their respective capsules and ligaments are set into motion and become flexible again. Pressure is gently and effortlessly put on the muscles running lengthwise to the spinal column concentrically and excentrically (tension toward and away from the body) equivalent to the physiological strain. The soft intervertebral discs are exposed to an alternating traction-compression-strain, which supports their enrichment with fluids and makes them suppler. The flowing movements cause a pump effect on the spinal fluid (liquor) that boosts its circulation. Setting in motion of the spinal column affects other regions of the body, too. After all the vertebral canal surrounds a large portion of the central nervous system, the nerve cords of the spinal marrow. This stimulus inevitably has to expand to the regions of the body supplied by the corresponding section of the spinal column. The vegetative nervous system is also stimulated because many of its tracts run a little in front of the spinal column into the depths of the torso. During the exercises the propioceptive nerve cells of all joints (they signal the joint's position to the brain) are constantly stimulated due to the changing pressure and constantly varying joint positions. All the body's joints are passively moved without being exposed to severe stretching. A psychological and physiological change takes place: psychological calming, lowering of the pulse and blood pressure. Warmth is spread. Some begin to sweat. Fingers swell. Sounds in the lower abdomen indicate an increased mobility of the gastro-intestinal tract. The autonomic nervous system is activated. The nervous activity increasingly switches from sympathetic to parasympathetic.

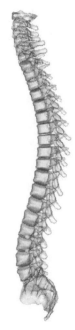

The whole spine, including sacrum and coccyx

The "waves on the ocean" exercise

The Qigong exercise, "waves on the ocean", is most suitable as an additional technique following the lumbar spine exercise. It is very effective for the entire spine.

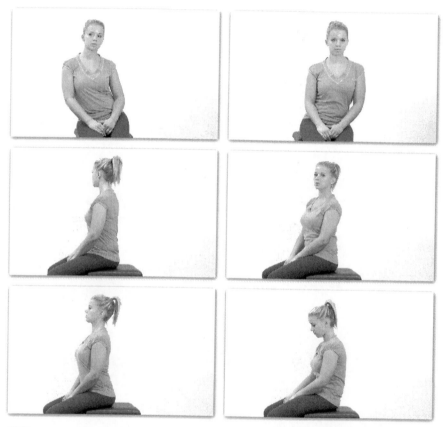

"Waves on the ocean", one of the oldest and most effective Qigong exercises

Sit in an upright and relaxed position on a chair or a stool and let your awareness sink to the lower end of your spine, to your sacral bone.

This exercise begins on the "maybe plane". Tilt your sacral bone slightly to the left (the sacral bone is just above the tailbone and below the last lumbar vertebra). Follow the spine's shifting to the left, one vertebra at a time, all the way to the head. Then you let the spine glide to the right in the same way. Do not exert yourself or try too hard. It suffices gently guiding your awareness to the area you want to move. When you repeat the movement, try to do so in an ever more fluid and faster motion. If you remain completely relaxed, you will fall into a quiet rhythm of movement that is like that of a snake. Maintain this movement until it feels smooth and your back muscles warm and loosen up.

If a particular section of your spine does not let itself be guided easily in one or the other direction, interrupt the exercise and do the following.

Test

Test whether the limited spine section can be guided comfortably in the opposite direction. If so, combine the movement with breathing. Is the movement more comfortable while breathing in or breathing out?

Exercise

Perform the combination of breathing and movement for several breaths.

Retest

Retest both directions of movement and be aware of any changes. If there is improvement, continue with the "waves on the ocean" exercise.

The "waves on the ocean" exercise can also be performed on both other planes. In the "yes plane", shift your tailbone slightly forwards. This causes the sacral bone and the entire pelvis to shift a little to the back. Then, without exerting yourself, shift all vertebrae from the bottom to the head backwards (caterpillar motion).

In the rotation ("no plane") the sacral bone and the tailbone turn together. Again, let all vertebrae follow from the bottom to the top (turning motion).

Option

In osteopathy "unwinding" refers to the untangling of the tissue. According to this technique, the self-treatment is performed as follows: After performing the exercises in the three planes separately, intuitively move out of the "no plane" into all planes simultaneously. Do this with playful ease and let yourself be guided by your feeling, as if watching your body move itself.

Unstable spine – "no plane"

Some spine problems are related to the instability of a segment of the spine. The spine has two different muscle systems: a global one, controlling all large movements of the entire body, as well as a local one, which stabilizes the spine. Imagine your spine to be a tower of building blocks or a tower of matchboxes. The global muscle system combines over large distances the bottom matchboxes with the top ones. The local system combines one box with the two neighboring ones. If something disturbs the tower's balance, the global system tenses on one side to maintain the balance. The local system, however, maintains the stability of the single segments. If there were no local system and the top and bottom box were pushed together, the boxes in between would be squashed out and the tower would collapse. The interaction of these two systems is extremely vital! The following exercises help to locate the loss of control of movement (instability) and to counteract it.

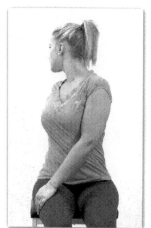 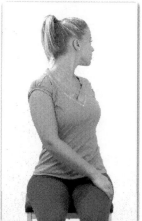

The pre-test is shown here. The actual exercise is performed without visible movements!

Test

Sit in an upright and relaxed position on a chair or a stool. Test the spine's rotation ("no plane") in both directions. While turning, be aware of the feeling in the lumbar spine and from when on the movement no longer is comfortable.

Now return to the initial position. Maintain part of your awareness in the problematic spine segment (often this is a segment of the lower lumbar spine) and imagine you are pushing your right knee forward. There should be no visible movement. The point is, that you get a feeling for controlling your muscles. You are testing the connection of your brain to your muscles. Return to the initial position and test the other knee, only in your imagination. If you can feel a distinct difference, this is probably due to a segmented instability. This might make itself noticeable by causing the feeling that many more muscles have to be utilized on one side while imagining the movement, while the other side feels like a well-functioning servomechanism. Sometimes the worse side even appears blocked. Have you detected which side is more comfortable (easier to control)? Then you just still need to find out which breathing phase best matches the movement.

Exercise

Perform the combination of breathing and movement for about two minutes. Maintain your awareness in the problematic segment. You do not require any anatomical knowledge for this. Simple feel the area. It might appear to outsiders that you have fallen asleep in a sitting position, even though, in reality, you have guided your awareness to the inside of your body and therefore are active indeed. Perform these exercises for segmented stabilization with particular inner awareness. It may take some time to obtain the desired results. Even discomforts that have existed for years have, in the case of most patients, improved after at least a month. Of course this requires daily exercise.

Retest

Retest both directions and be aware of any changes. Should it now be easier to steer towards the worse side, retest the spine's rotation like in the original test. You should perceive a significant improvement, as the two muscle systems' interaction is now more in tune.

Unstable spine – "maybe plane"

Test

Imagine you were trying to press one ischial tuberosity harder into the seat and be aware of the movement impulse. If you have instability problems, you will notice a difference when testing the other side. Which is the more comfortable direction? Which direction is easier to control? Now you only still need to match it to the right breathing phase.

Exercise

Perform the better combination of breathing and movement for approximately two minutes.

Retest

Retest and be aware of changes.

Exercise option on the "yes plane"

You should only test the "yes plane" after having done the exercises on the other planes several times or if you have so far not felt any differences.

Test

Imagine your pelvis were a bowl filled with water. Imagine you are tipping some of the water out the front. For the global muscle system, this would mean moving into an arching position, but no movement should be visible. Assess how easily you feel the impulse of movement. Now test the other direction. Imagine you are tipping some of the water out the back (causing the global muscle system to hunch your back). Test in your imagination how easily you can pull your pubic bone towards the tip of your sternum without actually moving. At the first impulse of movement in this direction you should feel your stomach muscles tensing slightly without contracting. Perform these tests playfully and without tensing up. Then assess whether one direction is easier or more comfortable than the other. Once you have decided which direction is more comfortable or easier controlled, match it to the right breathing.

Exercise

Perform the combination of breathing and movement for about two minutes.

Retest

Retest and be aware of changes

Support for the spine: from pelvis to feet

The next exercises focus on joints and muscles supporting the spine. They can provide back pain relief by keeping it in alignment and facilitating movements that extend or twist the spine. In Chinese medicine "strong legs" are essential to a relaxed and pain free back. So if a maladjustment in the areas mentioned below causes the spine to be off-balance, it automatically compensates, which can cause discomforts. If problems keep on and the spine exercises do not provide lasting relief, note in which other body areas you sense discomfort (onion of discomfort). Applying exercises to the corresponding area should reduce the discomforts in the back as well.

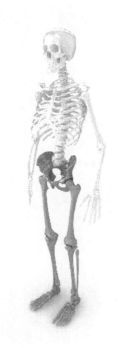

From pelvis to feet

Discomforts in the area of the pelvic floor

This exercise is suitable e.g. in support of a urinary incontinence therapy. It is also helpful in case of an unstable spine.

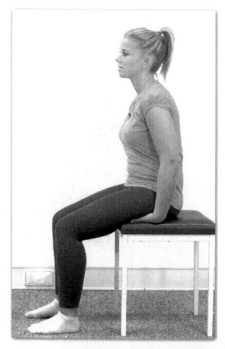

The pelvic floor exercise: gentle and effective

Test

Push the palms of your hands under your buttocks, so that the tips of your fingers can slightly grasp the ischial tuberosities.

Tense your pelvic floor. It might help imagining you are drawing your entire pelvic floor into yourself. See whether the tensing better matches breathing in or out. What counts, is the feeling of being able to control the muscles, not strength.

Exercise

Perform the combination of breathing and movement for at least two minutes. Pause your breathing for long enough to feel the inner impulse to continue breathing.

Retest

Retest you ability to control the muscles of your pelvic floor.

Discomforts in the area of the sacroiliac joint

This area is located to the left and right of the sacral bone.

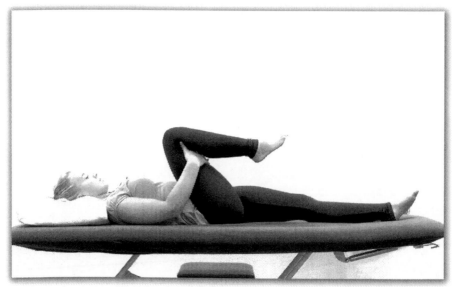

The sacroiliac joint exercise almost always has a positive effect, and often discomforts in that area are only the outer layer of the "onion of discomfort". So be mindful of any changes after the performance!

Test

Lie relaxed on a stable, but not too hard, surface. An exercise mat would be ideal. Lift your knee so far, that you can grab the hollow of your knee with your hands. If you are not able to do this, use a rolled-up towel to aid you. Be aware of how easy the movement is performed and how comfortable the final position is. Then test the other leg.

Exercise

Perform the exercise with the more comfortable side. Bend your leg and grasp the hollow of your knee with both hands.

During one breathing phase pull your leg slightly closer. During the other breathing phase move it back into the initial position. In most cases it is easier to pull the leg towards oneself while breathing in. Either way it should be completely relaxed. The movement stems from the arms and can be minimal. Perform the exercise for at least two minutes.

Retest

Retest the bending of both legs and be aware of any changes.

Discomforts in the gluteal area

The following exercise is loosely based on Dr. Johnston's "functional technique" and is wonderfully suited to the self-treatment of pain points in the gluteal area, which are often mistakenly labelled sciatica.

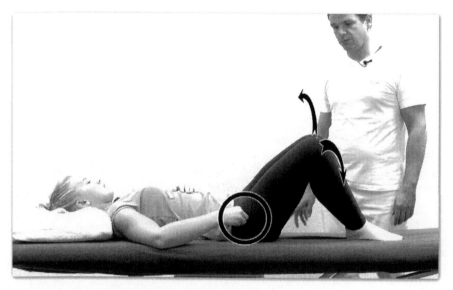

This exercise is helpful with discomforts from the gluteal area to the exterior part of the leg. It balances the pelvis.

Test

Lie on an exercise mat or on a similar surface and bend your knees with your feet remaining on the mat. Apply sufficient pressure to the pain point so that you can feel it. Hold this point and assess the tension and pain. Then slowly let the leg on the painful side fall to the outside.

Note how the tension and pain change in the point. Lift the leg back to the initial position. Now let the other leg slowly fall to the outside and take note of the pain point. Bring the leg back up to the initial position. Keep hold and take note of the point as you let both legs fall to the outside at the same time. Return to the initial position. Move both legs to the left, letting the knees and ankles touch. Afterwards move both legs to the right. One of these movements should clearly have reduced the pain and tension in the focused point. That is your exercise movement. Breathe in while moving into the more comfortable position, and out while returning to the initial position. Then switch the combination of breathing and movement, i.e breathe out while moving to the more comfortable position and breathing in while returning to the middle. Be gentle. You can often reach the most comfortable position with minimal movement.

Exercise

Perform the combination of breathing and movement with corresponding breathing pauses for several breaths.

Retest

Retest the pain point. Both pain as well as tension should be significantly reduced.

Option: During the exercise, remain in the most comfortable position and breathe in and out relaxed, not forgetting the breathing pauses.

Hip joint problems

The hip joint can be moved around all three movement axes. Usually the best results are achieved with exercises on the "no plane". You can perform the exercise lying down or standing up.

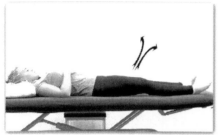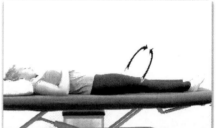

Rolling the legs to the outside and to the inside. The more gentle, the more effective!

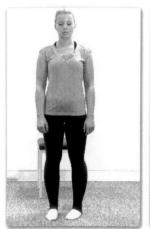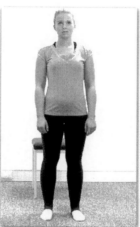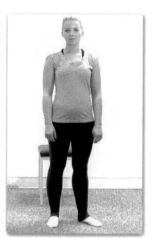

The exercise can also be performed standing

Test

Lie on your back and turn your right leg inwards/outwards. Test the left leg in the same way.

Which of the four movements is the most comfortable? Combine it with breathing. Is it best performed while breathing in or out?

Exercise

Perform the combination of breathing and movement for at least two minutes.

Retest

Retest all four directions of movement and be aware of any changes.

Option: Maintain the leg in the most comfortable position and breathe in and out relaxed. Do not forget the breathing pauses. This option is particularly suitable when performing the exercise standing up.

The area of the hip joint/pubic bone/adductors

The adductors are the muscles on your inner upper thigh. These are always tense with hip joint problems. Daily exercises over a prolonged period can be useful.

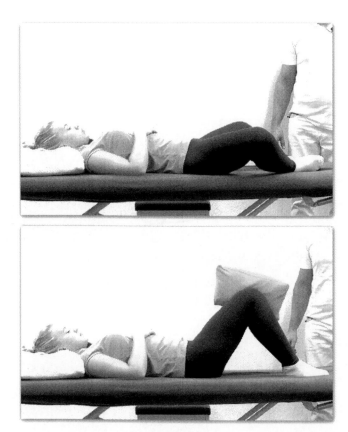

This exercise is also suitable for discomforts in the area of the pubic bone

Test

Bend your legs so that your knees create a 90-degree angle. Now slowly let your knees fall apart. As soon as you feel resistance, return to the initial position. Position your feet a little apart (30-40cm is usually the most comfortable) and press your knees together. Which position is more comfortable? If it is letting your knees fall apart then test whether it is best combined with breathing in or out. If you perceive the pressing together of the knees to be more comfortable, take a pillow or something similar, place it between your knees (the exercise can be performed without) and clasp it with your knees. Now test whether you can increase the pressure between your knees better while breathing in or while breathing out.

Exercise

Perform the most comfortable combination for at least two minutes.

Retest

Retest both options and be aware of any changes.

Knee exercise

Sit relaxed on a chair and place your hands, palms down, on your knees. Your feet are hip-wide apart and your ankles perpendicular to your knees.

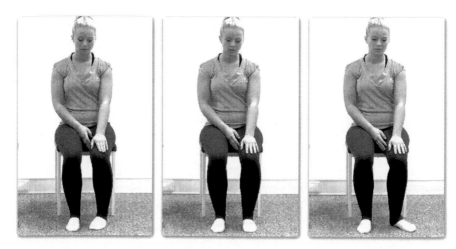

From left to right: foot turned inward, neutral and turned outward

Test

Turn your right foot to the inside. Maintain your leg's position and use your hands to stabilize your knee. Return to the initial position. Now turn your right foot to the outside. Now repeat the tests with your left foot. Which of the four directions is the most comfortable? Combine it with breathing. Does it better match breathing in or out?

Exercise

Perform the combination of breathing and movement for one to two minutes.

Retest

Retest all four directions and be aware of changes.

Exercise for the balance of the knee muscles

You need to test which of the three exercises is most effective for your knee.

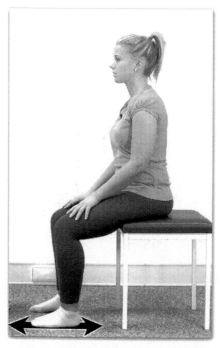

The illustrated movement is only imagined!

Test

Sit relaxed on a chair or a stool and gently press your feet into the floor. Place your hands on your upper thighs. Imagine moving your right foot forward. You will feel the muscles on the upper side of your upper thigh tense. Then imagine pulling your foot underneath the chair or stool. The muscles on the lower side of your upper thigh will tense. Which direction of tension is more comfortable? Then you only still need to find out whether it is best combined with breathing in or breathing out.

Exercise

Perform the combination for six to ten breaths.

Retest

Repeat the initial test and be aware of any changes.

Option 1: Test both legs at the same time by imagining pushing one foot away while pulling the other one under the chair or stool. Test how best you could combine breathing and tensing/relaxing your muscles.

Option 2: First test whether you can better turn your foot to the inside or to the outside and then maintain the better position. Then imagine pushing your foot away and pulling it towards you and perform the exercise with the more comfortable tension in the breathing rhythm.

Feet - Problems with the upper ankle joint

You will find a good exercise for feet in the chapter titled "headaches". The following exercises are best performed lying on your back.

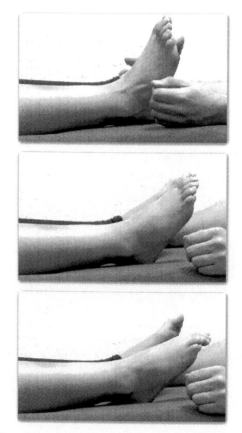

From left to right: toes pointing upward, neutral, pointing downward

Test

Test the feeling of pulling your toes towards you and stretching them away from you (movement on the "yes plane", bending/stretching in the upper ankle joint). Have you found a more comfortable direction of movement? Then you only still need to find out whether it is best combined with breathing in or breathing out.

Exercise

Perform the combination of breathing and movement for one to two minutes.

Retest

Retest both directions and be aware of changes.

Problems with the lower ankle joint

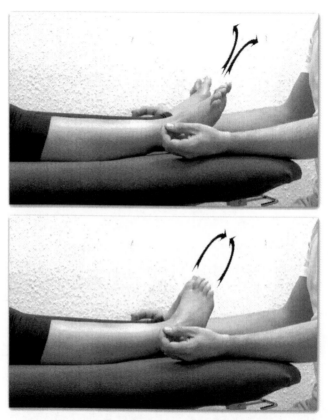

Feet turned away from each other, and the palms of the feet facing each other

Test

Test the feeling resulting from turning your ankles towards or away from one another ("maybe plane"). Have you detected a more comfortable direction of movement? Then you only still need to find out whether it is best combined with breathing in or breathing out.

Exercise

Perform the combination of breathing and movement for one to two minutes.

Retest

Retest both directions and be aware of any changes.

Shoulders

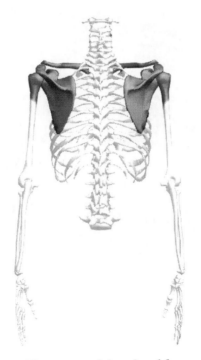

The area of the shoulders

Basic exercise for shoulder discomforts

If the following exercise does not provide any relief, try performing the next exercise for the acromioclavicular joint.

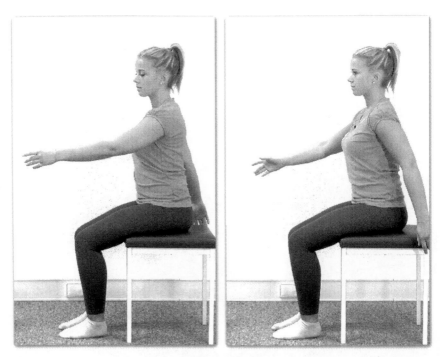

Arm movement as when walking

Test

Lift the left arm slowly, thumb pointing forward. Simultaneously, move the right arm to the back. Now the other way around: the right arm upward and the left arm to the back.

Have you found a more comfortable direction of movement? Now you only need to find out whether it is better combined with breathing in or breathing out.

Exercise

Perform the combination of breathing and movement for one to two minutes.

Retest

Retest both directions and be aware of changes.

Note: With acute discomforts, the amplitude of movement might be small. Please make sure you remain in your comfort zone.

This exercise takes place in the "yes plane". You can also perform the exercise on both other planes. On the "no plane" this means turning the affected arm to the inside/outside. One the "maybe plane" this means, stretching the arm sideways away from your body/pushing it sideways towards your body.

Dysfunctions in the area of the acromioclavicular joint

If you are suffering severe discomforts, this exercise should be performed lying on your back.

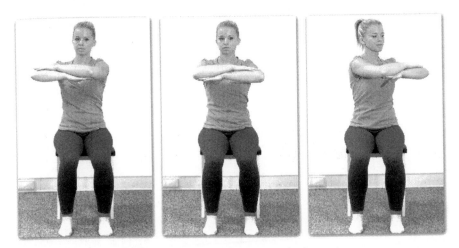

The "Kazachoc" (Cossack dance)

Test

Sit on a chair or a stool. Place your right underarm on top of your left underarm. Your chest, upper arms and underarms should form a rectangle. Without letting them break contact, move your underarms to the left. Be aware of a feeling of comfort while performing the movement, then return to the middle. Now place your left underarm on top of the right one and perform the movement to the right. Have you found a more comfortable direction of movement? Now you simply need to find out whether it is best combined with breathing in or breathing out.

Exercise

Perform the combination of breathing and movement for one to two minutes.

Retest

Retest both directions and be aware of changes.

"Grounding" and centering

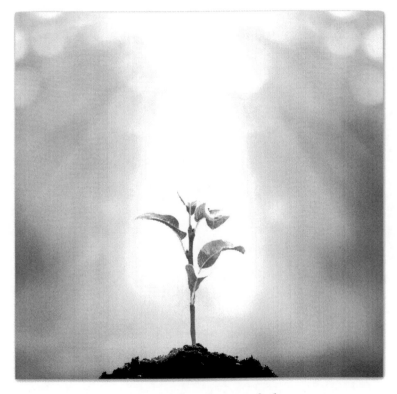

Centered and grounded

"Grounding" exercise

Bad feet can cause all kinds of back and hip and leg problems. Even in the case of headaches, it often makes sense to begin the treatment at your feet. You might know the proverb "Keep the head cool and the feet warm". The following exercise is particularly suitable if you are suffering of cold feet in addition to a headache. If you perform this exercise on a regular basis, you will notice a training effect: your feet will warm up ever quicker. And it will effect all areas between feet and head too.

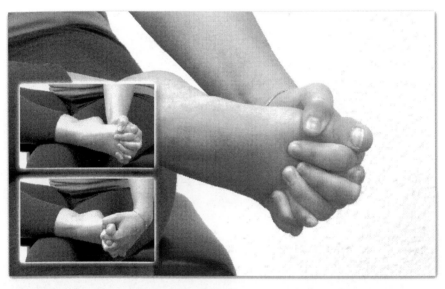

Not too easy but surprisingly effective every time: the toe exercise
Left: toes turned downwards and upwards

Test

Take your shoes and socks off and walk a few steps barefoot. Take note of the feeling in, and particularly under your feet. Now sit in a comfortable chair, although any chair will do the trick. Try grabbing your left foot with your right hand, interlinking your fingers with your toes so that your thumb and index finger are firmly grasping the big toe. Your index finger is between the big toe and the second toe. Try to stick your other fingers between your toes in the same manner.

You might have to practice this a few times. Should you not be able to stick your fingers between your toes, you can simply lay them on top and firmly grasp your foot. Is it easier to bend your toes upward or downward? Test whether the more comfortable direction is better combined with breathing in or breathing out.

Exercise

Repeat the most comfortable combination of breathing and movement for at least ten breaths. During the exercise, try to get your fingers as deep as possible between your toes in order to grasp your foot as firmly as possible. Just this once, it is okay if you feel a slight twinge.

Retest

Retest both directions and walk a few steps barefoot. You should be able to feel a clear difference in the sensation of the soles of your feet. This exercise alleviates the headache fairly quickly but your feet will probably only warm up after several hours.

Centering exercise

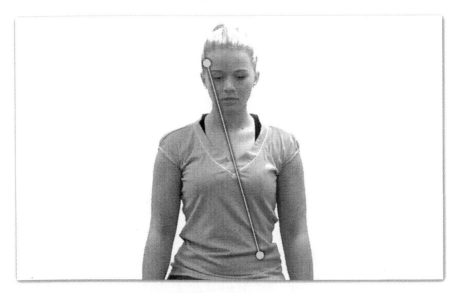

Connect the two points in your mind

Test

Test your inner balance. Stand with your feet shoulder-width apart and more or less parallel. Your knees should be minimally bent so that you can move your tailbone slightly to the front (straightening of the lumbar spine). Your spine is gently straightened; your head feels light and aims upward. In this position you feel a stronger pressure under your feet. Move your body weight onto your right foot and notice how far you can do this with ease. Then move back to the middle, pause and test the left side. Do both sides feel the same or are there differences? In the latter case, you should definitely try the following exercise.

Exercise

Remain in the position described in the test. Feet shoulder-width apart, your eyes gently closed or only slightly opened. Guide your awareness to your head. You will immediately perceive a point that draws your awareness to itself. This could be a tooth or a point on your skull, around your ear, etc. Gently take this point into your awareness and try to feel it precisely and to localize it. Where is it exactly? Now split your awareness: while being aware of the point, notice the ambient sounds (e.g. the ticking of a clock). Now guide your awareness to your body. You will straight away notice a second point. Be clearly aware of both points at the same time and in your mind connect them with a line. You could imagine this line to be a light beam, for instance. Maintain the focus of your awareness on this line and notice for several minutes what happens. If your thoughts drift, gently bring your awareness back to the line.

After some time the line appears to move towards the center of your body. But even if this does not occur, the exercise is effective. End it by stretching your knees, opening your eyes and shaking out your entire body.

Retest

Repeat the initial test and be aware of changes. How do you feel in general? Besides improving your inner balance, this exercise has a great effect on the vegetative nervous system, which among other things is also responsible for healing.

The idea for this exercise stems from a special area of osteopathy, in which we deal with "fulcrum techniques". A fulcrum is a center of rotation and pivot in the body, which the osteopath perceives with his hands. It corresponds with the line, which you could perceive in your body in this exercise. With help of the fulcrum techniques, the midline of your body is strengthened.

Exercise of the inner alchemy

"We find all of the parts of the whole solar system and the universe represented in man."

A.T. Still

The inner alchemy of antique, classic medicine deals with the training and cultivating of the spirit and psyche. The best-known exercise associated with it, is the so-called "small heavenly cycle", in which an inner movement, closely connected to your breathing, is performed. Its effect can be felt in the following exercise. At the outset of the book I asked you to notice a small stretching of your spine while breathing in. Now you will see that the opposite can happen.

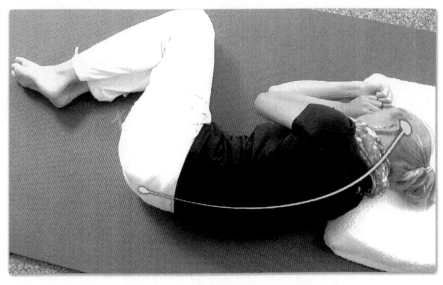

The central nervous system's key points of origin are mentally connected

Comfortably lie on your side in a fetal position. For several breaths be aware of the air flowing in and out of your nostrils. Now try to notice the air in the back of your nose, all the way into the nasopharyngeal space. Now imagine how the air travels into the area above your gums, i.e. between and behind your eyes. This is the area from which the body's central nervous system (brain and spinal cord) developed. Now place your middle- or index finger on the tip of your tailbone. Let your finger travel about 2-3 cm upward until you feel a small indentation. This is the lower end of the central nervous system. Maintain both these points in your awareness and in your mind combine them over your spine. It might help to imagine this connection as a glowing "C". When you breathe in, this "C" should bend more. When you breathe out it should straighten itself. This might be a very subtle movement, hardly noticeable from the outside. It is important that your imaginative powers remain in your body. This exercise has a strong effect on the vegetative nervous system, which means that after a few minutes you will feel very calm and relaxed.

Any questions?

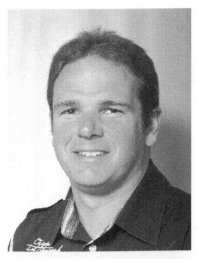

**Should you have any questions regarding the exercises,
or should you want to share experiences
or if you are interested in broadening your knowledge of osteopathic self-treatment in one of my seminars,
please visit my Facebook page:**

www.facebook.com/osteopathicselftreatment

Your Thomas Seebeck

Lotus-Press

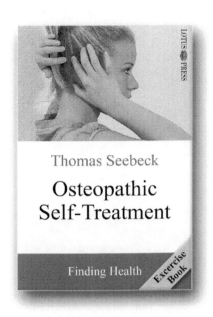

Thomas Seebeck
Osteopathic Self-Treatment: Finding Health

Osteopathy is on everyone's lips. In order to detect their patients' problems, osteopaths employ comprehensive skill and knowledge regarding the structure and function of the human body. A little-known fact, however, is that the osteopathic techniques and principles are wonderfully suited for self-treatment, as only the patient himself has a direct link to his inner self.

The first part of the book explains the principles of osteopathic treatment.

The book's main part is then the "osteopathic medicine cabinet" with 45 exercises for all areas of the body, from headaches to ankle sprains.

ISBN
- Paperback: 978-3-935367-19-4
- eBook: 978-3-935367-21-7
- eBook Kindle: 978-3-935367-20-0

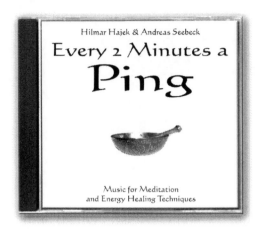

Hilmar Hajek & Andreas Seebeck

Every 2 Minutes a Ping - Music for Meditation and Energy Healing Techniques

A ping for every 2 minutes helps you to concentrate your thoughts into this healthy engagement exercise as the ping will bring your thoughts concentrated back into your meditation enabling you to take control of your mind, helping you remove those chains that binds you together with stress and depression. The music can be used to increase the effectivity for all forms of meditation practices or healing methods like Reiki, Jin Shin Jiutsu or the Healing Code. Try it now and see how effective it can be for you! Many have already tried it so why not grab that opportunity of being able to enjoy life to the fullest!

Compact Disk / mp3-download

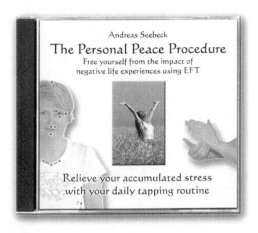

Andreas Seebeck
The Personal Peace Procedure - Free yourself from the impact of negative life experiences using EFT

Relieve your accumulated stress with your daily tapping routine.

The Personal Peace Procedure is your guide to learning the proper way on how to handle all the failures, stress and unhappy events of your life story for you to still be able to live a healthy and fit life despite the unfortunate circumstances in your life. Each of the segment is a crucial part in your healing of those hurtful feelings of the past. This procedure will help you move forward with your life and will help you see how lively it can be without weighing those negative feelings above your shoulders.

The Personal Peace Procedure uses the famous "Emotional Freedom Technique" by Gary Craig and is recommended to be done on a daily basis through identifying and resolving one problem at a time. This method has already been proven a success, so if you are one of those people who are still emotionally and psychologically distress with someone or something in the past, we recommend this method as the best way of helping you cut through those abusive ropes of misery that keeps you from seeing the beauty of what life has to offer.

Compact Disk / mp3-download

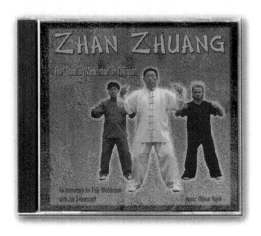

Jan Silberstorff
Zhan Zhuang

Zhan Zhuang is the Qigong exercise with the longest tradition which can be traced back 27 centuries. It is the foundation of all Qigong styles and is characterized by its great effectiveness and efficiency. For most people, training in Zhan Zhuang is a complete surprise in the beginning. There are no recognizable external movements, although it is a highly energetic exercise system. In contrast to many other methods, Zhan Zhuang develops our internal energy in a very efficient way, instead of consuming it. Zhan Zhuang Qigong is practiced in well-balanced standing positions which increase the flow of energy and build up internal strength. The Zhan Zhuang system is based on a unique fusion of relaxation and exertion which stimulates, cleanses and massages the whole body. Because Zhan Zhuang is so effective in raising our energy levels, it is often used as basic training for taijiquan.

Music: Hilmar Hajek

Tracks:
1. Instruction for beginners (22:00 min.)
2. Instruction for advanced pupils (40:00 min.)

Compact Disk / mp3-download

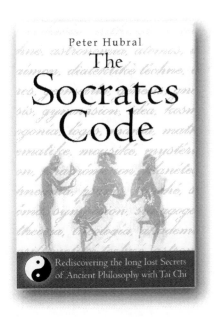

Peter Hubral

The Socrates Code: Rediscovering the long lost Secrets of Ancient Philosophy with Tai Chi

Peter Hubral sets out a meticulously researched and convincing case that Western Philosophy is founded less upon the original Ancient Greek texts, as on a careless and ahistorical misreading of them, for which he provides an unprecedented rigorous revision. Due matching the Dao-practice to the practice of dying, Hubral completely dismantles the illusion that the western world has constructed about Pythagoras, Socrates, Plato, etc. He shows that they made much more profound discoveries with the practice of dying about nature than what we are told about their contributions to mankind in uncountable commentaries!

ISBN
- Paperback: 978-1500465605 (also available as an ebook)

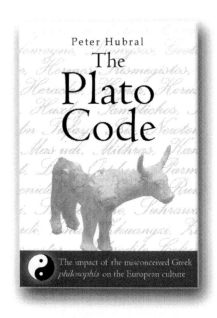

Peter Hubral
The Plato Code: The impact of the misconceived Greek philosophía on the European culture

The Plato Code extends The Socrates Code, which is the first book in a series of three, in which Peter Hubral dismantles today's understanding of the Pythagorean/Platonic philosophía, the mother of modern philosophy. He shows that its many Greek masters taught how to obtain extrasensory natural knowledge, which appears "out of itself" on what Lao Tzu calls in the Daodejing the Great Path (Da Dao) and Parmenides calls in his Poem on Nature the Path (Way) to Truth. This step-wise path from the known into the unknown provides pre-natal knowledge based on the unconditioned cognition principle: Consciousness can be significantly expanded by rigorous meditative dedication to Nothingness (Nonbeing). The composite lion-bull motive on the front cover is an ancient Iranian allegory for this principle. The philosophía can, like the Dao-teaching of Fangfu, only be understood with it.

ISBN
*   Paperback: 978-1500672249 (also available as an ebook)

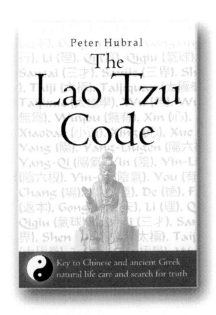

Peter Hubral

The Lao Tzu Code: Key to ancient Chinese and Greek natural life care and search for truth

Peter Hubral explains in detail the modern Tai Chi-teaching of Dao-grandmaster Fangfu which goes back to the Yellow Emperor and Lao Tzu. He demonstrates its excellent match with the written Greek Pythagorean/Platonic philosophía. He shows, how both teachings contribute to deepen the understanding of modern cognitive and health sciences as well as physical and psychic therapies. He provides with this inedited treatise on ancient Chinese wisdom a solid foundation for The Socrates Code, in which he completely revises the careless and ahistorical misreading of ancient Greek texts. He uses The Lao Tzu Code also to justify The Plato Code, in which he documents the strong impact that this misreading ironically had on the modern western culture.

ISBN
  •   Paperback: 978-1500821340 (also available as an ebook)

Lotus-Press recommends

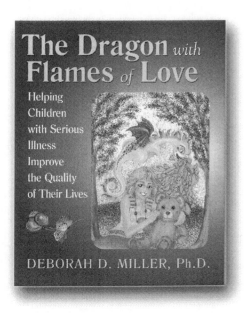

Deborah D. Miller, Ph.D.
The Dragon with Flames of Love

Deborah D. Miller, in her book "The Dragon with Flames of Love,"
is dedicated to empowering parents and children facing the challenge
of a serious illness. Her hands-on experience, the real-life examples
and the beautifully illustrated presentation provide a rich resource for
improving the quality of life of the child and loved ones coping with
the illness. In addition, her explanations of the highly effective tool
EFT (Tapping) and ways to support the child and family members
serve to educate and support anyone who is dedicated to helping children and their families. Deborah's wisdom, love and compassion are
felt throughout the book. She will inspire you as well as bring relief,
peace and hope. The Dragon with Flames of Love is truly a gift for
children and those who love them.

ISBN
- Paperback: 978-0976320067 (also available as an ebook)

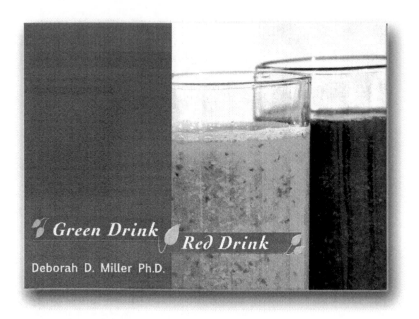

Deborah D. Miller, Ph.D.
Green Drink, Red Drink

Ever get frustrated with your weight or your health? You're probably not alone. In today's world of junk food and fast food, it is easy to make unhealthy choices. What is needed are simple and practical ways to consume health-providing foods. That is what this book is all about. It explains what you need, why it is important, how to create delicious and nutritious green drinks to supplement your diet, and it contains over 50 recipes for you to enjoy. Empower yourself to create the health you desire by adapting your daily intake to include more green drinks and red drinks. It is easy and fun as well as delicious-tasting. Deborah Miller's desire is to help people feel empowered and capable of maintaining a healthy state of mind and body. With a little knowledge and a few additions to one's eating regime, improvements can be made. This book is a great resource to help you along your way.

ISBN
• Paperback: 978-0976320043 (also available as an ebook)

For more information and
demo material visit us on
www.lotus-press.com

LOTUS **PRESS**

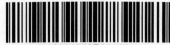

10901552R00065

Printed in Great Britain
by Amazon.co.uk, Ltd.,
Marston Gate.